I0767563

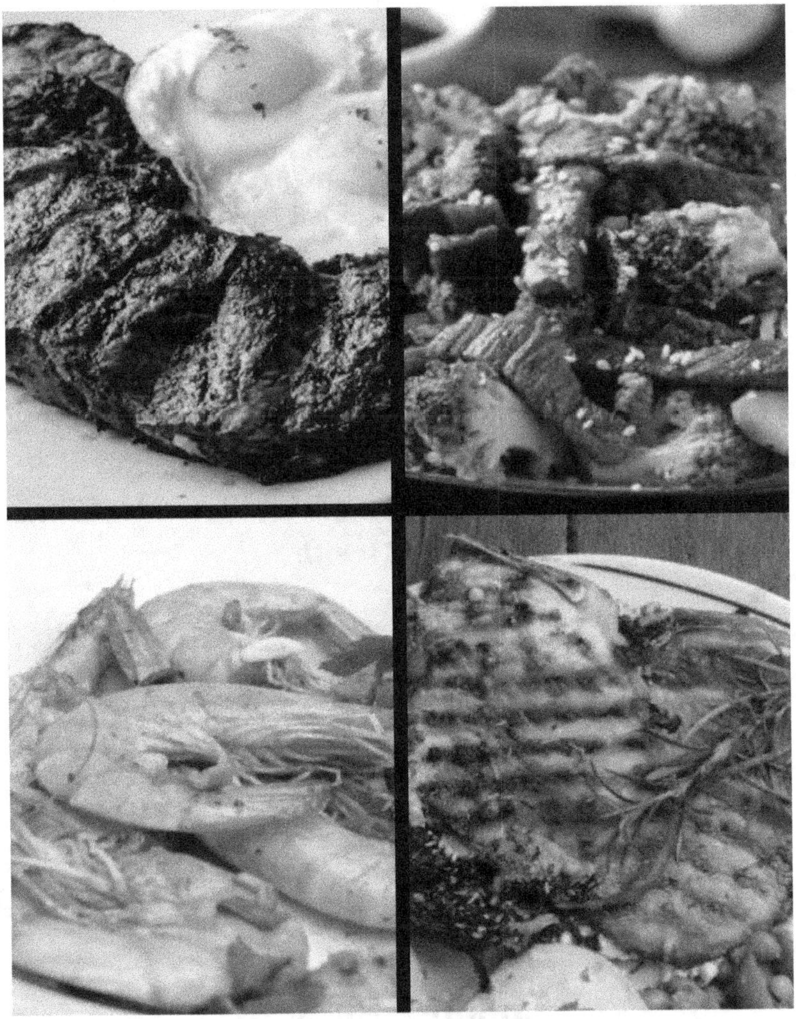

THE COMPLETE CARNIVORE DIET MEAL PLAN

The Ultimate Guide to Thriving on Animal-Based Eating for Weight Loss, Healing, and Health

By

Joanna Robbins

author disclaim all liability for any loss or damage resulting from or related to the use of this book.

The sole goal of this book is to be informative. The publisher and author do not provide any professional, legal, or medical advice. Should you need such guidance, please contact a qualified expert.

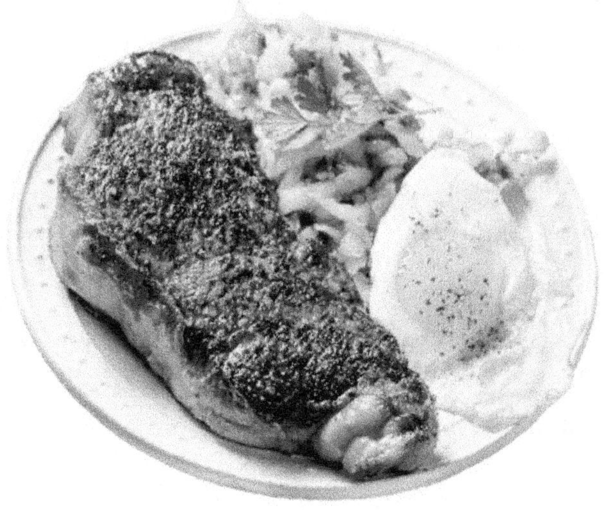

Table of contents

Introduction

The Carnivore Diet stands as a bold and contentious outlier. This dietary strategy promotes consuming only animal products and avoiding all plant-based meals, originating from a significant break from traditional beliefs. The Carnivore Diet has been more popular in recent years, attracting the interest of health enthusiasts, academics, and skeptics. Advocates highlight many possible advantages, including better digestion, higher energy levels, greater mental clarity, and weight reduction. Yet, despite the intense promotion, the Carnivore Diet remains cloaked in controversy and suspicion, with detractors voicing worries about possible nutritional inadequacies, environmental consequences, and the long-term sustainability of such an extreme eating pattern.

The Carnivore Diet is based on the eating patterns of early humans and hunter-gatherer societies, aiming to reconnect with our ancestral origins. Advocates claim that our pre-agricultural ancestors mostly survived on animal-based diets, flourishing on a nutrient-rich supply of meat, fish, and animal fats. They argue that humans have strayed from their natural dietary patterns only in recent centuries due to the rise of agriculture and the widespread use of processed foods. Advocates of the Carnivore Diet believe that returning to a diet focused on animal products may lead to maximum health and vitality, allowing individuals to recover their ancestral heritage.

"The Complete Carnivore Diet Meal Plan" emerges as a comprehensive guidebook for those daring to explore the realms of an exclusive animal-based diet. In a landscape rife with disinformation and opposing ideas, this book seeks to give clarity, advice, and practical tools for you as you begin your carnivore adventure. This book combines scientific evidence, practical guidance, and tasty recipes to clarify the Carnivore Diet, helping you make educated decisions about your dietary choices and health.

Within the pages of "The Complete Carnivore Diet Meal Plan," you will go on a voyage of exploration and discovery, diving deep into the subtleties of this controversial nutritional strategy. The book starts by establishing a strong base, exploring the historical origins and evolutionary background of the Carnivore Diet. From the dietary habits of our ancient ancestors to the scientific foundations supporting this atypical eating pattern, you obtain a detailed grasp of the Carnivore Diet's rationale and possible advantages.

As you journey deeper into the heart of the guide, you encounter practical advice and actionable strategies for implementing the Carnivore Diet in your daily life. From grocery shopping recommendations and meal preparation tactics to portion control techniques and dining out standards, this book offers you the skills and resources required to negotiate the obstacles and complexity of a meat-centric lifestyle. With specific sections for breakfast, lunch, and dinner, as well as a variety of tasty recipes and meal planning, you are taken step-by-step through the process of producing healthy and gratifying carnivore meals.

Yet, beyond the practicalities of meal planning and preparation, "The Complete Carnivore Diet Meal Plan" delves into the broader implications and considerations of adopting an exclusive animal-based diet. Addressing frequent misunderstandings and issues about the Carnivore Diet, you get insight into the nutritional adequacy, environmental effect, and ethical aspects of this eating strategy. Through a balanced exploration of the science, ethics, and practicality of the Carnivore Diet, you are empowered to make educated choices that correspond with your health, morals, and lifestyle objectives.

"The Complete Carnivore Diet Meal Plan" serves as a beacon of clarity and guidance in a sea of dietary confusion and uncertainty. Whether you are a staunch enthusiast, a curious skeptic, or somewhere in between, this book encourages you to go on a journey of self-discovery and change via the transformational power of food. As we travel together through the pages of this book, let us embrace the spirit of inquiry, open-mindedness, and investigation, as you unveil the secrets of maximum health and vigor on the Carnivore Diet.

Chapter 1

Getting Started with the Carnivore Diet

The Carnivore Diet, which excludes plant-based meals and only emphasizes animal products, has become more well-known in recent years due to its possible health advantages. But starting this gastronomic adventure calls for some planning and preparation. We'll cover all the essentials in this book, with a special emphasis on four areas: preparing your kitchen and pantry, setting realistic goals, assessing your readiness, and mental and emotional preparation.

Assessing Your Readiness

Determine if you're ready to make the switch to a carnivore diet before making any big dietary changes. This entails assessing a number of your present lifestyle, health, and mental state to make sure you're ready for any obstacles and changes that may arise from implementing this eating pattern.

1. Current Dietary Habits: Evaluate your diet and eating patterns at the moment. Do you usually eat a diet high in animal products, or do you also eat a lot of plant-based foods? Knowing where you are coming from will enable you to assess how big of a change switching to a carnivore diet could be.

2. Health Status: Take into account your present state of health as well as any potential medical issues. The carnivore diet has received a lot of attention because of its possible health advantages, but not everyone should follow it, particularly if they have specific medical issues. To determine if the carnivore diet is right for you, speak with a healthcare provider.

3. Commitment Level: Determine how dedicated you are to changing your diet. It takes commitment and self-control to follow a carnivore diet, especially in the beginning when your body may need some time to adjust to the new eating schedule. Assess your readiness to adhere to the food limitations and lifestyle modifications associated with the carnivore diet.

4. Knowledge and Preparation: Learn the tenets and recommendations of the carnivore diet. Learn about the kinds of foods that are permitted and prohibited on the diet, along with any possible advantages and disadvantages. Furthermore, think about whether you have access to the tools and networks that will assist your success, such as trustworthy suppliers of superior animal products and a group of people who share your nutritional philosophy.

Setting Realistic Goals

When beginning the carnivore diet, it is crucial to set reasonable and attainable objectives for yourself. Setting specific goals can help you remain motivated and focused throughout the process, which will make it simpler to monitor your development and make any required modifications as you go.

1. Health Goals: State precisely what health outcomes you want to get from a carnivore diet. These might include better digestion, more energy, weight reduction, or treatment for certain medical ailments. Set reasonable objectives based on your unique requirements and health situation, and think about speaking with a healthcare provider if you are unsure about what you can realistically achieve.

2. Dietary Goals: Establish your dietary objectives and preferences about the carnivore diet. Choose whether to adopt a strict carnivore diet that eliminates all plant foods or whether to include certain animal products, such as dairy or eggs. Establish guidelines for your daily food consumption, including portion sizes and macronutrient ratios, to make sure you're fulfilling your nutritional requirements and following the carnivore diet's tenets.

3. Behavioral Goals: Think about any adjustments you would need to make to your behavior to help you make the switch to a carnivore diet. This might include planning and cooking meals, purchasing foods that appeal to carnivores, or developing other coping mechanisms for stressful situations or emotional eating triggers. Establish concrete actions to assist you in bringing these changes about gradually and steadily over time.

4. Timeline: Set a reasonable deadline for yourself to meet your objectives and reach your benchmarks. Understand that incorporating a new eating style, such as the carnivore diet, into your daily routine may take some time. To stay responsible and motivated, set both short- and long-term objectives. However, be adaptable and ready to modify your schedule in light of your experiences and advancements.

<u>Preparing Your Kitchen and Pantry</u>

Getting your pantry and kitchen ready for the carnivore diet is crucial to making sure you have the supplies and foods you need to meet your nutritional objectives. You may reduce temptation and position yourself for success by clearing out things that don't fit the diet and filling your kitchen with carnivore-friendly meals.

1. Purge Non-Carnivore Foods: Start by eliminating any non-carnivore items from your kitchen and pantry, including grains, legumes, vegetables, fruits, and processed foods. This will help eliminate potential sources of temptation and guarantee that you're not tempted to depart from the carnivore diet.

2. Stock Up on Animal Products: The cornerstone of your carnivore diet should be made up of premium animal goods. Beef, pig, chicken, fish, eggs, and dairy products like cheese and butter may fall under this category. Whenever feasible, seek choices that are organic, wild-caught, grass-fed, or grown on pasture to optimize the density and quality of nutrients.

3. Include Nutrient-Dense Foods: You should think about including nutrient-dense foods such as organ meats, bone marrow, and bone broth in your diet in addition to animal products. The vital components included in these foods—vitamins, minerals, and amino acids—can promote general health and well-being when followed in conjunction with a carnivore diet.

4. Invest in Kitchen Tools: Stock your kitchen with necessary appliances and gadgets to streamline and expedite the process of preparing meals. A good chef's knife, cutting board, cookware, and gadgets for the kitchen—like an instant pot or slow cooker for making big quantities of meat—may be included in this.

Mental and Emotional Preparation

Making the switch to a carnivore diet takes mental and emotional preparation to overcome any obstacles and disappointments that may arise. You may increase your chances of long-term success on the carnivore diet by adopting a positive mentality and creating coping mechanisms for stress, cravings, and social pressures.

1. Mindset Shift: Be open-minded and ready to accept change while implementing the carnivore diet. Understand that your body may need some time to get used to the new eating schedule and that outcomes might not happen right away. Rather than concentrating on constraints or restrictions, consider the prospective health advantages and enhancements in well-being that you expect to accomplish with the carnivore diet.

2. Coping Strategies: As you go on your carnivore adventure, prepare yourself for whatever obstacles and temptations you may encounter. This might include finding alternative coping strategies for stress or emotional eating triggers, such as mindfulness training, engaging in physical activity, or contacting loved ones or online support groups.

3. Self-Reflection: To remain connected to your mission, take some time to consider why you chose to follow a carnivore diet. You should also periodically review your objectives. No matter how little, acknowledge and celebrate your accomplishments along the road, and take lessons from any failures or roadblocks you face. Instead of seeing these events as excuses to quit or lose hope, see them as chances for personal development and self-discovery.

4. Social Support: Be in the company of people who accept and understand your food choices. Tell others you know about your trip so they can support you, give you advice, and hold you accountable. Look for online forums, communities, or social media groups devoted to the carnivore diet to meet others who share your interests and share your experiences and perspectives.

Setting realistic objectives, organizing your pantry and kitchen, and developing the mental and emotional fortitude necessary to handle the ups and downs of this eating style are all necessary before beginning the carnivore diet. You may build a strong foundation for success and confidently and resolutely start your carnivore adventure by following these steps.

Chapter 2

The Science Behind the Carnivore Diet

The Carnivore Diet, characterized by its exclusive focus on animal-based foods and the complete exclusion of plant-based foods, has sparked significant interest and controversy within the realm of nutrition. The diet's proponents highlight its possible health advantages, while its detractors question its long-term viability and enough nourishment. We examine the science behind the carnivore diet in this thorough chapter, including understanding nutritional science, exploring health benefits, debunking myths and misconceptions, and evaluating research and evidence supporting the diet.

<u>Understanding Nutritional Science</u>

The basis for developing dietary guidelines is nutrition science. To assess the benefits and drawbacks of any dietary strategy, including the Carnivore Diet, one must have a fundamental understanding of nutrition.

1. Macronutrients and Micronutrients: Consuming macronutrients (proteins, fats, and carbs) and micronutrients (minerals and vitamins) forms the basis of nutrition. Meat, poultry, fish, and eggs are examples of animal-based meals that are a rich source of vital nutrients. These include complete proteins, important fatty acids, vitamins (including B12, A, D, and K2), and minerals (such as iron, zinc, and selenium). Determining the place of animal foods in a balanced diet requires an understanding of their nutritional makeup.

2. Bioavailability and Absorption: An important benefit of eating animal-based meals is their high bioavailability or the body's ease of absorbing and using the nutrients. For instance, animal proteins help produce hormones, support immunological function, and aid in muscle regeneration by containing all the required amino acids in the ideal ratios for human health. Similar to this, the body absorbs iron and zinc from animal sources more easily than from plant ones.

3. Potential Nutritional Gaps: Although meals derived from animals are rich in vital nutrients, questions have been raised about possible nutritional gaps in the Carnivore Diet. For instance, a diet lacking in plant foods may have a decreased intake of antioxidants, phytonutrients, and dietary fiber—all of which are crucial for immune system function, digestive health, and the prevention of illness. To maximize the nutritional sufficiency of the Carnivore Diet by deliberate meal selections and supplements, it is important to comprehend these possible gaps.

Exploring the Health Benefits

The Carnivore Diet's proponents tout its possible health advantages, which include less inflammation, better metabolic health, weight reduction, and more mental clarity. Even though the majority of the data behind these assertions is anecdotal, a new study indicates that the Carnivore Diet may have some positive health effects.

1. Weight Loss and Metabolic Health: One of the Carnivore Diet's most often mentioned advantages is its capacity to encourage weight reduction and enhance metabolic health. The Carnivore Diet has the potential to cause ketosis, a metabolic state in which the body burns fat for fuel, by removing carbs and substituting protein and fat for energy. Reduced appetite, enhanced satiety, and greater insulin sensitivity have all been linked to ketosis, and these effects may help with weight reduction and metabolic enhancements.

2. Mental Clarity and Cognitive Function: A few people claim that the Carnivore Diet improves their mental clarity and cognitive performance. Although the exact processes causing this occurrence are unknown, steady blood sugar levels, decreased inflammation, and optimal brain fuel usage have all been suggested as potential contributors. Furthermore, anecdotal evidence indicates that food factors including gluten and lectins may be avoided to reduce symptoms of brain fog and enhance general cognitive performance.

3. Reduced Inflammation and Autoimmune Conditions: Chronic inflammation is linked to the development of several illnesses, including arthritis, cardiovascular disease, and autoimmune disorders. It has been shown that meals derived from animals, especially those high in antioxidants and omega-3 fatty acids, have anti-inflammatory qualities. Further study is required to clarify the underlying processes and long-term consequences of the Carnivore Diet, however, some people report improvements in inflammatory indicators and symptom control of autoimmune disorders.

Debunking Myths and Misconceptions

The Carnivore Diet has been met with skepticism and condemnation in equal measure, with critics voicing worries about the diet's nutritional suitability, possible health hazards, and environmental effects. Understanding the subtleties of the Carnivore Diet and making educated dietary selections need the ability to distinguish reality from myth.

Myth: The Carnivore Diet Lacks Essential Nutrients

A prevalent misperception about the Carnivore Diet is that it does not include every vital nutrient required for optimum well-being. Although plant-based meals do add to total nutritional consumption, animal-based foods provide a great source of vitamins, minerals, vital fatty acids, and complete proteins. The Carnivore Diet may be nutritionally sufficient with proper planning and supplements if needed.

Myth: The Carnivore Diet Is Unsustainable and Environmentally Harmful

The Carnivore Diet's detractors often claim that it is unsustainable and harmful to the environment since it emphasizes meals derived from animals. There are sustainable and regenerative farming methods that put animal welfare, soil health, and ecosystem integrity first, even though industrial animal agriculture does have a major negative influence on the environment. Furthermore, proponents of the Carnivore Diet contend that mono-crop agriculture, which mostly depends on chemical inputs and leads to soil degradation and biodiversity loss, may have a larger environmental impact than well-managed ruminant agriculture.

Myth: The Carnivore Diet Is Unsafe and Unhealthy

The possible health dangers associated with the carnivore diet, such as malnourishment, cancer, and cardiovascular disease, are cited by critics. While it's true that there are hazards associated with any diet, the Carnivore Diet may be safe and beneficial to health for certain people when followed correctly. Furthermore, newer studies indicate that the Carnivore Diet may provide special therapeutic advantages for several medical diseases; nevertheless, further investigation is required to completely comprehend the diet's long-term implications.

Research and Evidence Supporting the Carnivore Diet

Although anecdotal evidence predominates in the Carnivore Diet's support, a growing corpus of scientific studies is examining the diet's possible health benefits and underlying causes. A preliminary study indicates that certain components of the Carnivore Diet may provide therapeutic advantages for a range of medical ailments, but additional research is required to make firm findings.

1. Metabolic Health and Weight Loss: Several studies have looked at how low-carb, high-protein diets—which are comparable to the Carnivore Diet—affect weight loss and metabolic health. Compared to traditional low-fat diets, research indicates that low-carb diets may result in more weight reduction, better insulin sensitivity, and positive changes in blood lipid profiles. These results suggest that the Carnivore Diet may be beneficial for controlling weight and maintaining metabolic health, but further studies are required to fully understand its long-term impacts.

2. Autoimmune Conditions and Inflammation: New research indicates that nutritional therapies, such as the Carnivore Diet, may be therapeutically effective in treating inflammation and autoimmune diseases. It has been shown that meals derived from animals, especially those high in antioxidants and omega-3 fatty acids, have anti-inflammatory qualities. Low-carb, high-protein diets have been linked to improvements in inflammatory indicators and symptom management of autoimmune diseases, including inflammatory bowel disease and rheumatoid arthritis. To validate these results and comprehend the processes behind the reported impacts, additional study is necessary.

3. Gut Health and Digestive Disorders: Research is now being conducted to determine how nutrition affects gut health and digestive problems. Plant-based diets are often marketed for their high fiber content and possible advantages for gut bacteria; nevertheless, some people may have digestive problems, including gas, bloating, and pain in the abdomen, after ingesting certain plant foods. The elimination of potentially irritating plant chemicals, known as the Carnivore Diet, may provide relief for those suffering from digestive diseases. However, more study is necessary to fully comprehend the impact of this diet on gut microbiota and long-term gastrointestinal health.

The science behind the Carnivore Diet is complex and multifaceted, encompassing aspects of nutritional science, health benefits, myths and misconceptions, and research evidence. While anecdotal evidence predominates in the diet's support, new research indicates that certain elements of the carnivore diet may have therapeutic advantages for a range of medical ailments. To completely comprehend its long-term consequences and implications for health and well-being, further study is necessary.

Chapter 3

Transitioning to the Carnivore Diet

Transitioning to the Carnivore Diet represents a significant dietary shift that requires careful planning, preparation, and support. Even though the diet has many potential advantages, going through the transition period may be difficult for the body and the mind. In this chapter, we explore key aspects of transitioning to the Carnivore Diet, including managing transition symptoms, tips for a smooth transition, and common challenges to help individuals navigate this transformative journey with confidence.

Managing Transition Symptoms

As the body adjusts to a new nutritional paradigm, switching to a carnivore diet may cause a variety of physical and psychological symptoms. Minimizing pain and maximizing the transition process need an understanding of these symptoms and good management strategies.

1. Common Transition Symptoms: Although they differ from person to person, common transition symptoms include headaches, exhaustion, lightheadedness, gastrointestinal problems (like constipation or diarrhea), cravings, mood changes, and irritability. These symptoms often appear as the body becomes used to not having carbs and starts to depend more on fat and protein for energy.

2. Hydration and Electrolyte Balance: It's critical to keep these two aspects of your health in check throughout the changeover period. Eliminating carbs may increase the excretion of electrolytes and water, which may result in electrolyte imbalances and dehydration. Make sure you are getting enough water and electrolytes (sodium, potassium, and magnesium) from foods and supplements such as mineral-rich water and bone broth.

3. Gradual Reduction of Carbohydrates: Before completely switching to the Carnivore Diet, some people may find it helpful to lower their carbohydrate consumption gradually. This strategy may lessen the feelings of withdrawal linked to carbohydrate restriction and help make the switch to a mostly animal-based dietary pattern easier.

4. Patience and Persistence: Throughout the transition period, practice self-compassion and patience. It's common to feel uncomfortable and to have difficulties while adjusting to a new dietary regimen. Remind yourself of the possible rewards that lie ahead after the transition time and have faith in the process.

Tips for a Smooth Transition

A meticulous approach to planning, preparing, and executing the Carnivore Diet is necessary for a successful transition. A more seamless and easier transition to the new diet plan may be achieved by including the following advice in your plan of action.

1. Educate Yourself: Invest some time in educating yourself with the fundamentals, possible advantages, and typical drawbacks of the Carnivore Diet. You'll be better able to make judgments and handle the transition process by knowing the science and reasoning behind the diet.

2. Gradual Elimination of Plant Foods: Rather than making drastic dietary adjustments, think about progressively cutting down on and removing plant-based items from your diet. By using this strategy, the intensity of the transition symptoms is reduced and your body may gradually get used to not having carbs.

3. Focus on Nutrient-Dense Animal Foods: During the transition period, give top priority to foods that are high in nutrients, such as meat, chicken, fish, eggs, and organic meats. As you adjust to the Carnivore Diet, these items enhance general health and well-being by supplying critical nutrients in their most accessible forms.

4. Experiment with Meal Timing and Composition: Determine what works best for you by experimenting with various meal timing and composition techniques. While some people do well with smaller, more frequent meals, others prefer to have two or three bigger meals each day. Recognize your hunger signals and modify the time and makeup of your meals appropriately.

5. Listen to Your Body: Pay attention to the cues your body gives you and modify your eating plan appropriately. Observe how various meals and eating habits impact your mood, digestion, energy level, and general well-being. To ensure that your transition to the Carnivore Diet goes as smoothly as possible, follow your gut and adjust as necessary.

Common Challenges and How to Overcome Them

Making the switch to a carnivore diet comes with several obstacles that might impede development and drive. Achieving long-term success and diet adherence requires acknowledging these obstacles and putting plans in place to address them.

1. Social Pressure and Judgement: Social pressure and criticism from friends, family, and peers is a major obstacle experienced by those making the switch to the Carnivore Diet. Those who follow standard dietary rules may be skeptical of and critical of the diet due to its unorthodox character. To get beyond this obstacle, concentrate on convincingly explaining the Carnivore Diet to others and sharing its possible advantages with them. Be in the company of people who appreciate your nutritional choices and who will encourage you along the journey.

2. Cravings and Food Withdrawal: Cravings for comfort foods may surface when the body gets used to not having carbs and switches to using fat and protein instead. As people cut out processed and addictive foods from their diet, they may also suffer symptoms of food withdrawal. Animal meals high in nutrients that satisfy and satiate are the best way to beat cravings and food withdrawal. Try varying the cooking times and flavorings of your food to make it more palatable. To discern between genuine hunger and cravings, engage in mindful eating and pay attention to your body's signals of fullness and hunger.

3. Digestive Disturbances: Making the switch to a carnivore diet may momentarily impair digestive processes, resulting in symptoms like gas, bloating, constipation, or diarrhea. These symptoms often appear when food composition and fiber consumption varies, causing the gut flora to adapt. Prioritize electrolyte balance and hydration, eat enough animal fats, and gradually increase your consumption of organ meats and bone broth—foods that promote gut health and integrity—to relieve digestive difficulties. To support a balanced and healthy population of gut bacteria, think about including foods high in probiotics, including fermented dairy products or supplements.

4. Lack of Variety and Boredom: Eating only animal-based meals is said to result in a lack of diversity and a sense of culinary ennui, which presents another difficulty for those following the carnivore diet. Embrace imagination and experimentation in the kitchen to conquer this issue by experimenting with various meat cuts, cooking methods, and taste combinations. Include a variety of animal products, such as fish, chicken, beef, eggs, and organ meats, to provide enough nutrients and a pleasing texture. Carnivore-friendly cookbooks, internet sites, and discussion boards may be great places to find new recipes and meal concepts that fit your dietary needs and objectives.

Transitioning to the Carnivore Diet is a transformative journey that requires careful planning, preparation, and support. Through the appropriate management of transition symptoms, the use of transition-planning advice, the resolution of common obstacles, and the utilization of support networks and resources, people may confidently traverse the transition process and attain sustained success and contentment on the Carnivore Diet.

Chapter 4

Levels of Carnivore Eating

The carnivore diet is often perceived as a strict dietary regimen that excludes all plant-based foods. However, there is a range of carnivore eating styles within the carnivore group, each with unique subtleties and variances. By being aware of these various degrees of carnivore eating, people may adjust their diet to suit their tastes, objectives, and dietary requirements.

Different Approaches to Carnivore Eating

1. Strict Carnivore: Also referred to as the "zero-carb carnivore" or "all-meat diet," the "strict carnivore" strategy is at the most stringent end of the range. This method places a strong emphasis on eating only meals derived from animals—no plant foods at all. Strict carnivores usually steer clear of fruits, vegetables, grains, legumes, and processed meals, and instead concentrate on meats such as beef, hog, chicken, fish, eggs, and dairy products.

2. Low-Carb Carnivore: Unlike strict carnivore diets, the "low-carb carnivore" strategy permits some flexibility in the number of carbohydrates consumed, however, it is still far lower than recommended by most dietary standards. Low-carb carnivores acquire most of their calories and nutrients from animal-based meals, although they may sometimes eat modest quantities of low-carb plant foods including leafy greens, cruciferous vegetables, and certain herbs and spices.

3.   Carnivore-Adjacent: A "carnivore-adjacent" diet combines aspects of carnivore feeding with other dietary guidelines or limits. This is a strategy that some people choose to follow. Carnivore concepts may be included in eating habits while allowing for certain non-carnivore foods, such as those who follow a paleolithic diet (based on foods thought to have been eaten by early humans) or a ketogenic diet (high-fat, low-carb).

4. Modified Carnivore: The "modified carnivore" strategy is tailoring the carnivore diet to each person's requirements, preferences, and situation. This might include experimenting with varied macronutrient ratios (protein, fat, and carbohydrates), including "flexible" days or occasional cheat meals when non-carnivore items are permitted, or modifying the length and frequency of carnivore phases within a larger nutritional framework.

Zero-Carb Carnivore vs. Low-Carb Carnivore

1. Zero-Carb Carnivore: These animals consume just animal products; they do not allow any carbs to come from plants in their diet. This strategy seeks to reduce insulin response, enhance fat metabolism, and get rid of any allergies or irritants that could be present in plant-based diets. Fatty meats, organ meats, and animal fats are usually prioritized by zero-carb carnivores to satisfy their energy and dietary demands.

2. Low-Carb Carnivore: Low-carb carnivores permit a certain amount of carbohydrate consumption, but it is still much less than suggested by traditional dietary guidelines. While each person may have a different threshold for carbs, low-carb carnivores often place a higher value on foods rich in fat and protein and low in carbohydrates, such as dairy products, eggs, and fatty meat cuts. This strategy may maintain the metabolic advantages of carbohydrate restriction while allowing for more freedom in meal planning and food selection.

Incorporating Variety in Your Diet

Despite what is often believed, a carnivore diet may provide a surprisingly wide range of food alternatives, enabling people to tailor their meals to suit their tastes and dietary objectives. Adding diversity to your carnivore diet guarantees a better-balanced intake of vital minerals and micronutrients, as well as increased gastronomic delight.

1. Animal Protein Sources: To add variety to your carnivore diet, investigate several kinds of animal protein sources. Beef, hog, chicken, fish, shellfish, game meats, and organ meats are a few examples of this; each has a distinct taste, texture, and nutritional makeup. Try a variety of meat cuts, cooking styles, and flavor blends to make your meals tasty and engaging.

2. Fats and Oils: To provide necessary fatty acids and improve taste and satiety, include a range of healthful fats and oils into your carnivore diet. Choose plant-based fats like avocado, coconut, and olive oil as well as natural sources of animal fats like tallow, butter, ghee, and fatty meat cuts. To give your meals depth and richness, use a variety of fats in your cooking and meal preparation.

3. Organ Meats and Offal: When preparing your carnivore meals, don't ignore the nutritional powerhouse that is organ meats and offal. One of the foods that is highest in nutrients is organ meat; it contains a variety of vitamins, minerals, amino acids, and bioactive substances that are necessary for optimum health and vitality. Try liver, heart, kidney, brain, and other organ meats to experience the whole range of nutritional advantages they provide.

4. Eggs and Dairy Products: To add diversity and adaptability to your meals, include eggs and dairy products in your carnivore diet. Dairy items like cheese, yogurt, and cream give more protein, fat, and taste to eggs, which are a nutrient-dense source of high-quality protein, vitamins, and minerals. For the best nutritional density and quality, choose full-fat, pasture-raised, and organic choices wherever feasible.

<u>Finding Your Optimal Level</u>

To get the ideal balance of sustainability, health, and enjoyment, you must experiment with various methods, pay attention to your body's signals, and modify your dietary decisions as necessary. There's no one-size-fits-all method when it comes to carnivore eating, and what suits one person may not suit another. To discover what suits you best on your carnivore journey, it's important to be flexible and open-minded.

1. Self-Experimentation: Investigate various degrees of carnivore feeding by taking a proactive stance toward self-experimentation and self-discovery.

Observe how your body reacts to different meals, meal combinations, and eating schedules. Take note of any changes in your mood, digestion, energy levels, or general state of health. To record your findings and spot trends over time, maintain a food journal or diary.

2. Bio-individuality: Be aware that your ideal degree of carnivore eating may vary according to your unique genetics, metabolism, lifestyle, and health. It's important to tailor your strategy to your requirements and circumstances since what works for one person may not work for another. Be prepared to modify your eating habits and choices as necessary to better suit your priorities and objectives.

3. Listen to Your Body: Acquire the skill of paying attention to your body's signs and signals about hunger, fullness, desires, and contentment. Consider the physical, mental, and emotional effects of various meals on you. Utilize this knowledge to influence your meal planning and food selections. When it comes to providing your body with the nourishment it needs on a carnivore diet, follow your gut and intuition.

4. Consult with a Professional: For individualized advice and help in determining your ideal degree of carnivore diet, think about speaking with a trained nutritionist or healthcare professional. A skilled professional may assist in evaluating your unique objectives, food preferences, and state of health as well as provide evidence-based advice catered to your particular requirements. Develop a sustainable, well-rounded carnivore eating plan that promotes your general health and well-being by collaborating with your healthcare team.

Exploring the different levels of carnivore eating allows individuals to customize their dietary approach to suit their preferences, goals, and nutritional needs. Whether you stick to a modified, low-carb, or pure carnivore diet, finding your ideal degree of carnivore eating and integrating variety may improve your pleasure of food, help long-term carnivore lifestyle adherence, and support metabolic health. You may successfully navigate your carnivore path by practicing self-experimentation, bio-individuality, listening to your body, and getting expert help when necessary.

Chapter 5

Planning Your Carnivore Meals

Adopting a carnivore diet requires careful planning and preparation to ensure that you're meeting your nutritional needs while enjoying a varied and satisfying array of meals. Planning and preparing your carnivore meals may be made easier by concentrating on important details like grocery shopping, meal prep, and portion management.

<u>Grocery Shopping for Success</u>

The cornerstone of a good carnivore diet's meal planning is grocery shopping. You may equip your kitchen with the essentials needed to make satisfying and fulfilling carnivore meals by choosing high-quality, nutrient-dense animal products and basic ingredients.

1. Prioritize Animal Protein: Make a range of cuts and varieties of meat, poultry, fish, and shellfish your main focus while making your shopping list. Whenever feasible, choose organic, wild-caught, grass-fed, pasture-raised, or organic choices to optimize nutritional density and reduce exposure to detrimental additions or pollutants.

2. Include Organ Meats and Offal: When procuring carnivore components, do not undervalue the nutritional potency of organ meats and offal. Add organ meats (liver, heart, kidney, and brain) to your meal rotation to supplement important vitamins, minerals, and amino acids that muscle meat alone may not deliver.

3. Select Quality Fats and Oils: To improve the taste and nutritional value of your carnivore meals, use high-quality fats and oils. To provide vital fatty acids and encourage satiety, use plant-based fats like avocado, coconut, and olive oil, as well as animal fats like butter, ghee, tallow, and lard.

4. Opt for Whole Foods: Make sure to choose whole, minimally processed foods to get the most nutrients and to reduce your exposure to artificial substances, preservatives, and additives. Whenever feasible, go for fresh, unprocessed cuts of meat, poultry, and fish instead of processed deli meats or convenience meals.

5. Stock Up on Staples: To improve the taste of your meals without adding calories or carbs, keep your pantry well-stocked with important carnivore essentials like salt, pepper, herbs, and spices. Try a variety of spices and taste combinations to add novelty and enjoyment to your carnivore diet.

6. Plan for Variety: To make your meals interesting and fulfilling, try to include a range of animal protein sources, meat cuts, and cooking techniques on your grocery list. To guarantee a balanced intake of vital nutrients and avoid meal boredom, alternate between various cuts of meat, poultry, and seafood each week.

7. Consider Budget and Convenience: When creating your carnivore grocery list, consider your lifestyle and financial constraints. When looking for ways to save costs without sacrificing quality, look for ways like purchasing in bulk, taking advantage of bargains and promotions, and choosing canned or frozen meats and seafood.

8. Read Labels Carefully: When buying processed or packaged carnivore foods like sausage, bacon, or canned fish, be sure to thoroughly read the labels to look for chemicals, fillers, and hidden sugars that may not be in line with your diet. Whenever feasible, look for items with few ingredients and no artificial chemicals or added sugars.

Meal Prep Tips and Strategies

The key to effectively following a carnivore diet is meal planning. It will help you save time, reduce stress, and make sure you always have wholesome meals accessible throughout the week. The process of organizing, cooking, and enjoying your carnivore meals may be made more efficient by implementing effective meal prep techniques and ideas into your daily routine.

1. Batch Cooking: Set aside time every week to cook in bulk big amounts of animal protein and basic ingredients that may serve as the basis for many meals. Large roasts, entire chickens, or quantities of ground beef may be prepared ahead of time and then portioned into individual meals that can be warmed up and enjoyed all week long.

2. Pre-Portion Meals: To simplify meal preparation and portion management, divide cooked meats and other carnivore foods into portion-sized containers or resealable bags. Meals may be quickly and conveniently grabbed on the go, at work, or home when they are proportioned.

3. Prep Ingredients Ahead of Time: To save time and effort while putting meals together, wash, cut, and prepare vegetables, herbs, and other ingredients beforehand. To preserve freshness and guarantee that prepared items are accessible when required, store them in the refrigerator in airtight resealable bags or containers.

4. Utilize Slow Cookers and Instant Pots: To make meal preparation and cooking on a carnivore diet easier, make use of slow cookers, pressure cookers, and other kitchen equipment. While an Instant Pot can swiftly cook meats and other ingredients to perfection in a fraction of the time, a slow cooker is ideal for simmering bone broth, braising tougher types of meat, or cooking big quantities of stews and soups.

5. Plan for Leftovers: Accept leftovers as a useful and easy method to eat carnivore meals all week long. To generate leftovers that may be used as-is for simple and fast lunches or dinners, or as ingredients for new meals, cook additional amounts of meat and other carnivore-friendly items.

6. Experiment with Meal Components: To keep your carnivore meals intriguing and fulfilling, be inventive when it comes to meal components and taste combinations. Try varying the meat cuts, cooking techniques, spices, and sauces to liven up your meals and make them more exciting without sacrificing nutritional value or following the carnivore diet.

7. Schedule Meal Prep Sessions: To guarantee consistency and effectiveness in the planning and preparation of your carnivore meals, set aside a certain time each week for meal prep sessions. Meal planning should be prioritized alongside other crucial responsibilities and chores in your calendar to ensure consistency and momentum in your carnivore journey. Treat it like a non-negotiable appointment.

Understanding Portion Control

When following a carnivore diet, portion management is essential to controlling calorie consumption and making sure you're getting enough nutrients. You can maintain balance and moderation in your carnivore meals without overindulging or undereating by learning portion management concepts and putting them into practice in your meal planning and eating habits.

1. Focus on Protein: Make items high in protein your main focus while preparing carnivore meals, and try to have a substantial amount of animal protein at each meal. Protein is the foundation of a healthy, well-balanced carnivore diet because it supports satiety, metabolic function, and muscle development and repair.

2. Consider Fat Intake: When organizing carnivore meals, keep in mind that fat is a rich source of calories that may make a big difference in your total energy consumption. Although fat is an important part of a carnivore diet and offers useful nutrients and energy, it's crucial to control portion sizes to avoid consuming too many calories.

3. Monitor Hunger and Satiety: When following a carnivore diet, pay attention to your body's signals of hunger and satiety to help you choose how much food to eat and when. Instead of feeling too full or constrained, eat until you are pleasantly content. Also, observe how various meals and meal combinations impact your energy levels, appetite, and desires.

4. Use Visual Cues: To determine the right serving amounts for meals that carnivores, use visual cues and standards for portion proportions. Aim to have a fist-sized quantity of non-starchy veggies or other low-carbohydrate meals on your plate, a thumb-sized portion of fat, and a palm-sized portion of protein. Feel free to vary portion sizes according to your activity level, hunger, and personal tastes.

5. Practice Mindful Eating: On a carnivore diet, use mindful eating practices to improve portion management and foster a healthy connection with food. Rather than eating more out of habit or boredom, take your time, slow down, and enjoy every mouthful, paying attention to the flavor, texture, and other sensory aspects of your food. Stop when you're full.

6. Adjust Portion Sizes as Needed: Be adaptable and prepared to change portion sizes to your unique requirements, objectives, and situation. A calorie deficit may be achieved by gradually reducing portion sizes if your goal is to lose weight or change your body composition. On the other hand, those who need more energy or who engage in more physical activity could require bigger amounts to meet their demands.

7. Track Progress and Adjust Accordingly: To measure your progress and pinpoint areas for improvement, keep a record of your meal composition, portion sizes, and total amount of food consumed. To ensure that your carnivore diet is successful, monitor your adherence to portion control rules over time by recording your meals and using tools like food diaries, tracking apps, or portion control guidelines. Make modifications as necessary.

Planning your carnivore meals involves careful consideration of grocery shopping, meal prep, and portion control to ensure that you're meeting your nutritional needs while enjoying delicious and satisfying meals. You may make meal preparation and execution of carnivore meals easier by emphasizing high-quality animal protein, using effective meal prep techniques, and exercising conscious portion management. This will support your carnivore lifestyle and promote health and pleasure.

Chapter 6

Essential Nutrients on the Carnivore Diet

The carnivore diet is centered around animal-based foods, which provide a rich source of essential nutrients necessary for optimal health and well-being. A person on a carnivore diet may make sure they're fulfilling their nutritional requirements and following the guidelines of the diet by giving priority to nutrient-dense animal proteins, lipids, and micronutrients.

Protein

Protein is the cornerstone of the carnivore diet, providing essential amino acids necessary for muscle growth, repair, and overall metabolic function. Because animal proteins have all nine necessary amino acids—which the body cannot manufacture on its own and must get from diet—they are regarded as complete proteins.

1. Muscle Maintenance and Repair: Protein is necessary for those on a carnivore diet, especially for those who exercise or do strength training since it plays a critical role in promoting muscle development and maintenance. Consuming enough protein aids in the maintenance of lean muscle mass and facilitates the healing of muscles damaged by exercise.

2. Satiety and Appetite Regulation: Protein is a highly satiating food, which means that it may assist with feelings of fullness and satisfaction. This can help with appetite control and weight management while following a carnivore diet. Meals and snacks that are high in protein may help suppress cravings, cut down on snacking, and encourage diet adherence.

3. Metabolic Function: Protein's role in metabolism includes the synthesis of hormones, the generation of enzymes, and the maintenance of the immune system. On a carnivore diet, adequate protein consumption promotes good metabolic function, energy generation, and general health and vigor.

4. Sources of Protein on the Carnivore Diet: A wide range of foods, including fish, poultry, eggs, dairy products, beef, hog, and poultry, are high in animal proteins. Including a variety of animal proteins in your diet guarantees that you are getting the right amount of each of the necessary amino acids and supports adequate nutrition overall.

Fats

Fats are a primary source of energy in the carnivore diet, providing a concentrated source of calories and essential fatty acids necessary for various physiological functions. Saturated and monounsaturated fats, which are abundant in animal fats in particular, are essential for maintaining cellular structure, hormone synthesis, and food absorption.

1. Energy Production: In a carnivore diet, fats are a rich supply of energy that power metabolic activities, physical exertion, and day-to-day living. Fats are a crucial part of a low-carb, high-fat diet because, unlike carbs, which are restricted on the carnivore diet, they may be digested for energy even in the absence of glucose.

2. Brain Health and Cognitive Function: Because the brain is mostly made of fatty acids and needs a consistent supply of dietary fats to operate at its best, fats are essential for both brain health and cognitive function. A carnivore diet that includes sufficient levels of healthy fats promotes mood stability, memory, and cognitive performance.

3. Cellular Structure and Integrity: Fats are essential parts of cell membranes, giving all of the body's cells structural support and integrity. On a carnivore diet, consuming enough fat guarantees the preservation of healthy cell membranes, which are necessary for the transportation of nutrients, the elimination of waste, and general cellular function.

4. Sources of Fats on the Carnivore Diet: Animal fats may be found in a variety of foods on a carnivore diet, including fatty meat cuts, chicken skin, organ meats, bone marrow, and dairy products like butter and cheese. To bring more diversity and taste to carnivore meals, plant-based fats like avocado, coconut, and olive oils may be used in moderation.

Micronutrients and Supplements

While foods derived from animals are a great source of vital nutrients, a carnivore diet may be deficient in certain micronutrients, therefore it's important to pay close attention to nutrient intake and consider supplementing to avoid deficits.

1. Vitamins and Minerals: Vitamin B12, vitamin D, iron, zinc, and selenium are among the many vitamins and minerals found in animal proteins and lipids. These nutrients are necessary for the synthesis of red blood cells, the immune system, and healthy bones, among other physiological processes. However, the carnivore diet limits plant-based sources of vitamins and minerals, such as fruits, vegetables, and grains, which might result in shortages if not properly handled.

2. Supplementation: To guarantee nutritional sufficiency and avoid deficiencies, people on a carnivore diet may find it helpful to take supplements of certain micronutrients. Vitamin D, magnesium, omega-3 fatty acids (EPA and DHA), and electrolytes including salt, potassium, and magnesium are often suggested supplements on the carnivore diet. Furthermore, if a person's diet isn't providing enough iron or zinc, they could need to take supplements.

3. Bio-availability: Vitamins and minerals derived from animals are usually more bioavailable—that is, the body can absorb and use them more easily—than those derived from plants. On the carnivore diet, people may optimize the bioavailability of vital nutrients and reduce the need for supplements by concentrating on nutrient-dense animal foods.

4. Individual Variability: Age, sex, activity level, heredity, and health state are some of the variables that might affect an individual's nutrient needs. To find the right supplement plan for your unique situation, it's critical to evaluate your nutritional requirements and speak with a trained nutritionist or healthcare provider.

Essential nutrients on the carnivore diet include protein, fats, vitamins, and minerals necessary for optimal health and well-being. Individuals who follow a carnivore diet may make sure they're fulfilling their nutritional demands and benefit from this particular dietary strategy by emphasizing nutrient-dense animal proteins and fats and considering supplements as required.

Chapter 7

The Carnivore Diet Meal Plan

The carnivore diet, characterized by the consumption of primarily animal-based foods while excluding plant-based foods, has gained popularity for its potential health benefits and simplicity. When following the guidelines of the diet, a well-crafted carnivore meal plan offers a framework for satisfying satiety, maximizing health, and fulfilling nutritional demands. We examine a range of carnivore breakfast, lunch, and dinner alternatives in this chapter, providing you with scrumptious and fulfilling dishes to help you on your carnivore journey.

Breakfast

Breakfast on the carnivore diet often consists of protein-rich foods that provide sustained energy and promote satiety throughout the morning. Start your day with a substantial carnivore breakfast with a variety of alternatives, ranging from robust meat-based meals to easy egg recipes.

1. Classic Bacon and Eggs

Ingredients:

- Bacon strips

- Eggs

Preparation:

1. In a skillet, cook bacon until crispy.

2. Crack eggs into the same skillet and heat until done.

2. Steak and Eggs

Ingredients:

- Steak cuts (such as filet mignon, sirloin, or ribeye)

- Eggs

Preparation:

1. Use salt and pepper to season the meat.

2. Cook the steak on a grill or pan-sear it to your desired doneness.

3. Eggs may be cooked as desired or sunny-side up.

4. Place the eggs on the side of the heated steak.

3. Sausage Patties with Scrambled Eggs

Ingredients:

- Sausage patties

- Eggs

Preparation:

1. In a skillet, fry sausage patties until they are browned and well-cooked.

2. Scramble eggs in another skillet until they are set.

3. Serve scrambled eggs with hot sausage patties.

4. Egg and Bacon Breakfast Muffins

Ingredients:

- Bacon slices

- Eggs

Preparation:

1. Set oven temperature to 175°C/350°F.

2. Place bacon pieces in the muffin tray to create a cup shape.

3. In each bacon cup, crack one egg.

4. Bake the eggs for 15 to 20 minutes, or until set.

5. As muffins, serve hot.

5. Ham and Cheese Omelette

Ingredients

- Ham slices, diced

- Eggs

- Cheese (cheddar or your choice)

Preparation:

1. Cook chopped ham in a pan until it starts to become golden.

2. After beating the eggs, cover the ham in the skillet.

3. Top the eggs with cheese.

4. Keep cooking until the cheese melts and the eggs are set.

5. After folding, serve the omelet hot.

6. Egg and Sausage Breakfast Casserole

Ingredients:

- Sausage links, cooked and sliced

- Eggs

- Cheese

Preparation:

1. Preheat the oven to 375°F, which is 190°C.

2. Line the bottom of a baking dish with grease and arrange the cooked sausage pieces.

3. Pour beaten eggs over sausage.

4. Top with cheese, if desired.

5. Bake for 25 to 30 minutes, or until cheese is browned and eggs are set.

6. Warm casserole pieces should be served.

7. Bacon Wrapped Breakfast Sausages

Ingredients:

- Breakfast sausages

- Bacon slices

Preparation:

1. Wrap each breakfast sausage with a strip of bacon.

2. If necessary, fasten with toothpicks.

3. Cook the sausages through and the bacon crisp on the grill or in the oven.

4. Serve hot for a high-protein breakfast choice.

8. Egg and Chorizo Breakfast Burrito

Ingredients:

- Chorizo sausage, cooked

- Eggs

- Low-carb tortillas (optional)

Preparation:

1. In a skillet, scramble eggs until done.

2. Reheat the prepared chorizo in the same skillet.

3. If using, spoon chorizo and eggs onto tortillas, then fold them into burritos.

4. Warm-up and savor.

9. Egg and Cheese Breakfast Muffins with Sausage

Ingredients:

- Sausage links, cooked and chopped

- Eggs

- Cheese

Preparation:

1. Grease a muffin tray and preheat the oven to 350°F (175°C).

2. Combine cheese and cooked sausage in each muffin cup.

3. Pour beaten eggs over the combination of cheese and sausage.

4. Muffins should bake for 20 to 25 minutes to set.

5. Serve hot for a quick and easy breakfast choice.

10. Turkey Bacon and Egg Cups

Ingredients:

- Turkey bacon slices

- Eggs

Preparation:

1. Preheat the oven to 375°F, which is 190°C.

2. To make cups, line a muffin tray with pieces of turkey bacon.

3. In each bacon cup, crack one egg.

4. Bake the eggs for 15 to 20 minutes, or until set.

5. As individual egg cups, serve hot.

Lunch

Lunchtime on the carnivore diet offers an opportunity to enjoy a variety of protein-rich dishes that provide sustained energy and satisfaction to power you through the afternoon. There are several options for delectable and filling carnivore meals, ranging from hearty meat salads to aromatic seafood dishes.

1. Grilled Chicken Caesar Salad

Ingredients:

- Chicken breast

- Romaine lettuce

- Caesar dressing

Preparation:

1. Use pepper and salt to season the chicken breast.

2. Cook the chicken completely on the grill.

3. The grilled chicken should be sliced and served over romaine lettuce.

4. Enjoy after drizzling with Caesar dressing.

2. Beef Burger Lettuce Wraps

Ingredients:

- Ground beef

- Lettuce leaves

- Optional toppings: cheese, bacon, pickles

Preparation:

1. Make patties out of ground beef and cook them on a grill or pan fry until they are cooked through.

2. Fold the big lettuce leaves around the burger patties.

3. If desired, add the optional toppings.

4. As lettuce wraps, serve.

3. Steak Salad with Blue Cheese Dressing

Ingredients:

- Steak cuts (such as strip loin or ribeye)

- Mixed greens

- Blue cheese dressing

Preparation:

1. Steak may be pan-seared or grilled to the desired doneness.

2. Place thinly sliced steak over mixed leaves.

3. Add a blue cheese dressing drizzle.

4. As a substantial steak salad, serve.

4. Carnivore Pizza with Pepperoni and Cheese

Ingredients:

- Ground beef or pork (for crust)

- Pepperoni slices

- Cheese (mozzarella or your choice)

Preparation:

1. On a baking sheet, press ground beef into a thin crust.

2. Cook the crust in the oven until it's fully done.

3. Place cheese and pepperoni slices on top of the baked crust.

4. Put the cheese back in the oven and let it become bubbling and melted.

5. Serve hot as a pizza fit for a carnivore.

5. Grilled Lamb Chops with Mint Sauce

Ingredients:

- Lamb chops

- Fresh mint leaves

- Olive oil

Preparation:

1. Season lamb chops with salt and pepper after rubbing them with olive oil.

2. Chops of lamb should be grilled until done.

3. Blend fresh mint leaves with olive oil to make mint sauce.

4. Present the grilled lamb chops beside a serving of mint sauce.

6. Tuna Salad Stuffed Avocado

Ingredients:

- Canned tuna

- Avocados

Preparation:

1. After draining, combine tuna in a can with olive oil or mayonnaise.

2. Halve the avocados and remove the pits.

3. Place tuna salad into avocado halves.

4. Serve as a wholesome and revitalizing lunch choice.

7. Turkey and Cheese Roll-Ups

Ingredients:

- Sliced turkey breast

- Sliced cheese (cheddar or your choice)

Preparation:

1. Place a piece of cheese on each of the flattened turkey slices.

2. Roll up the cheese-filled turkey pieces.

3. If necessary, fasten with toothpicks.

4. Serve as a straightforward, high-protein lunch.

8. Beef Stir-Fry with Vegetables

Ingredients:

- Beef strips (such as sirloin or flank)

- Assorted vegetables (bell peppers, onions, broccoli)

- Soy sauce (optional)

Preparation:

1. In a heated skillet, stir-fry the beef strips until browned.

2. Stir-fry the mixed veggies until they become crisp-tender.

3. If desired, add soy sauce for seasoning.

4. Serve hot for a filling and healthy midday meal.

9. Chicken Wings with Hot Sauce

Ingredients:

- Chicken wings

- Hot sauce

- Butter (optional)

Preparation:

1. Bake or fry chicken wings until they are cooked through and crispy.

2. Add wings to spicy sauce (and melted butter, if preferred, for extra richness).

3. Serve hot for a spicy and tasty midday meal.

10. Salmon Fillet with Lemon Butter Sauce

Ingredients:

- Salmon fillet

- Butter

- Lemon juice

Preparation:

1. Sprinkle salt and pepper on the salmon fillet.

2. Bake or grill fish until it's done.

3. Melt butter in a small pot and stir in lemon juice.

4. Pour cooked salmon with lemon butter sauce.

5. Squeeze in a fresh lemon and serve hot.

<u>Dinner</u>

Dinner on the carnivore diet offers a chance to enjoy a variety of flavorful and satisfying meat-based dishes that provide essential nutrients and promote satiety. There is a limitless variety of tasty and healthy meat-based meal options, from tender steaks to hearty stews.

1. Ribeye Steak with Garlic Butter

Ingredients:

- Ribeye steak

- Butter

- Garlic cloves

Preparation:

1. Use salt and pepper to season the ribeye steak.

2. The steak may be seared or grilled to the appropriate doneness.

3. Melt butter and chopped garlic in a small pot until fragrant.

4. Before serving, brush the grilled steak with garlic butter.

2. Pork Chops with Rosemary Infusion

Ingredients

- Pork chops

- Fresh rosemary

- Olive oil

Preparation:

1. Season pork chops with salt and pepper after rubbing them with olive oil.

2. Cook the pork chops until done by grilling or pan-frying them.

3. Before serving, garnish with fresh sprigs of rosemary.

3. Bacon-Wrapped Chicken Thighs

Ingredients:

- Chicken thighs

- Bacon strips

Preparation:

1. Use salt and pepper to season the chicken thighs.

2. Tent each thigh of chicken with a bacon strip.

3. Cook the chicken on the grill or bake it until the bacon crisps up.

4. Grilled Lamb Kabobs

Ingredients:

- Lamb cubes

- Red onion chunks

- Bell pepper chunks

Preparation:

1. Lamb cubes are threaded onto skewers in succession with bits of onion and bell pepper.

2. Cook the lamb on the grill until it reaches the desired doneness and the veggies become soft.

5. Pan-seared duck Breast with Cherry Sauce

Ingredients:

- Duck breasts

- Cherries

- Red wine (optional)

Preparation:

1. Score duck breast skin and season with salt and pepper.

2. Duck breasts should be pan-seared skin side down until the skin is crispy.

3. Cook until done, flipping once.

4. Reduce and thicken the sauce by simmering pitted cherries in red wine.

5. Place on top of duck breasts.

6. Grilled Salmon with Dill Butter

Ingredients:

- Salmon fillets

- Butter

- Fresh dill

Preparation:

1. Use salt and pepper to season the salmon fillets.

2. Cook the fish on the grill until it's done.

3. Add finely chopped fresh dill to melted butter.

4. Before serving, drizzle some dill butter over the cooked fish.

7. Beef Short Ribs with BBQ Glaze

Ingredients:

- Beef short ribs

- BBQ sauce

Preparation:

1. Use salt and pepper to season the beef short ribs.

2. Bake or grill until thoroughly done.

3. Cook the ribs for a few minutes more, then brush them with BBQ sauce.

8. Pan-seared tuna Steaks with Lemon Pepper

Ingredients:

- Tuna steaks

- Lemon zest

- Black pepper

Preparation:

1. Sprinkle black pepper and lemon zest over tuna steaks.

2. Sear tuna steaks by pan-searing them in a hot skillet until the exterior is pink and the inside is seared.

9. Carnivore Stir-Fry with Beef and Broccoli

Ingredients:

- Beef strips (such as flank or sirloin)

- Broccoli florets

- Soy sauce (optional)

Preparation:

1. In a heated skillet, stir-fry the beef strips until browned.

2. Stir-fry the broccoli florets until they become crisp-tender.

3. If desired, add soy sauce for seasoning.

10. Grilled Shrimp Skewers with Garlic Butter

Ingredients:

- Shrimp

- Butter

- Garlic cloves

Preparation:

1. Assemble shrimp using skewers.

2. Shrimp skewers should be cooked thoroughly and pink on the grill.

3. Before serving, melt butter and chopped garlic, then brush the shrimp with it.

A well-designed carnivore meal plan offers a variety of delicious and satisfying options for breakfast, lunch, and dinner that provide essential nutrients and promote satiety while adhering to the principles of the diet. By including a varied variety of protein-rich meals, healthy fats, and tasty ingredients, those following a carnivore diet may enjoy a balanced and nutritious approach to eating that promotes their health and well-being.

Chapter 8

Optimizing Performance and Fitness on the Carnivore Diet

Achieving peak performance and optimal fitness on the Carnivore Diet requires more than just dietary adherence—it demands a strategic approach to exercise, recovery, and lifestyle habits. We explore the relationship between physical activity and the Carnivore Diet in this in-depth analysis, providing athletes, fitness enthusiasts, and energetic people with useful advice, methods, and recommendations. This manual offers a step-by-step plan for maximizing fitness and performance on the Carnivore nutrition, covering everything from striking the ideal balance between nutrition and exercise to improving muscle development and recovery.

Carnivore Diet and Exercise

Exercise and the demands of the Carnivore Diet must be carefully balanced, taking into account each person's unique objectives, food choices, and metabolic changes. This section looks at ways to follow the Carnivore Diet's tenets while incorporating exercise into a carnivore lifestyle, maximizing energy, and reaching performance objectives.

1. Fueling Workouts with Animal Protein and Fat: On the Carnivore Diet, exercise performance depends on getting enough animal protein and fat to maintain muscular function and give long-lasting energy. Prioritize meals high in protein, such as eggs, fish, chicken, and beef, both before and after exercise to aid in muscle regeneration and repair. While exercising, include wholesome fat sources like butter, tallow, and fatty meat cuts to boost energy and encourage fullness.

2. Adjusting to Metabolic Adaptations: Making the switch to a carnivore diet might require physiological adjustments that impact energy levels and exercise capacity. People may have changes in energy metabolism, glycogen storage, and electrolyte balance in the early stages of dietary transition. These changes may affect their ability to exercise and how hard they feel. Give your body enough time to acclimate to the Carnivore Diet, and then modify the length and intensity of your workouts to account for changes in your metabolism.

3. Tailoring Exercise Programming: To maximize performance and reach fitness objectives, exercise programming must be customized to follow the Carnivore Diet's tenets. To maintain lean muscle mass and increase strength, concentrate on resistance training. Compound exercises like squats, deadlifts, and bench presses work for numerous muscular groups at once. Shorten the length of aerobic exercise sessions by including sprint intervals and high-intensity interval training (HIIT) to improve metabolic conditioning and cardiovascular fitness.

Enhancing Recovery and Muscle Growth

To promote optimum performance and adaptability, recovery and muscular growth—which are crucial components of fitness—require attention to lifestyle variables, sleep patterns, and diet. This section looks at ways to maximize the health advantages of exercise, support long-term fitness performance, and improve muscle development and recovery while following a carnivore diet.

1. Prioritizing Protein Intake: Because it contains the essential amino acids required for tissue synthesis and repair, protein is vital for muscular development and recuperation. Make protein consumption your top priority after working out to take advantage of the anabolic window that occurs after exercise, which will aid in muscle protein synthesis and recuperation. To optimize muscle repair and adaptation, try to have a high-quality animal protein source, such as beef, poultry, or fish, for a protein-rich supper or snack during the first hour after an exercise session.

2. Supporting Nutrient Repletion: Micronutrients, electrolytes, and glycogen reserves are all depleted during exercise and must be replenished to promote performance and recuperation. To regain hydration and mineral balance after exercise, concentrate on rehydrating with electrolyte-rich liquids like bone broth or electrolyte-enhanced water. Add items rich in carbohydrates, such as fruit or honey, to your post-workout meals to help your body rebuild glycogen reserves and aid in recovery, especially after lengthy or intense workouts.

3. Optimizing Sleep and Stress Management: Sleep and stress reduction are essential elements of recuperation and adjustment, impacting immunological response, hormone balance, and physical performance. Make great sleep your priority by sticking to a regular sleep schedule, setting up a calming nighttime ritual, and improving the sanitation and surroundings of your sleeping space. Use techniques for reducing stress, such as deep breathing exercises, mindfulness meditation, and recreational activities, to lessen the negative effects of stress on healing and to enhance general well-being.

Tips for Athletes and Active Individuals

A customized approach to training, nutrition, and recuperation is necessary for athletes and active persons who are pursuing ambitious fitness objectives while following the Carnivore Diet. These individuals confront unique obstacles and possibilities. This section provides useful advice and techniques for maximizing performance, energizing exercises, and reaching the pinnacle of athletic performance while following a carnivore diet.

1. Monitor Hydration Status: Exercise performance and general health depend heavily on being hydrated, especially while following the Carnivore Diet, which might change electrolyte and fluid balance. Before and after exercise, keep an eye on your level of hydration by monitoring your body weight changes, urine color, and thirst signals. To stay hydrated and boost exercise performance, drink plenty of fluids throughout the day, including electrolyte-rich drinks like bone broth or electrolyte-enhanced water.

2. Experiment with Pre-Workout Nutrition: Exercise performance, energy levels, and perceived effort may all be impacted by a pre-workout diet, so it's important to try out a variety of approaches to see which one suits your requirements the best. While some people may find that working out while fasting is preferable, others may find that having a modest, high-protein breakfast or snack before working out helps to enhance muscular function and give sustained energy. Try varying pre-workout meal times, types, and amounts to maximize results and improve training responses.

3.   Prioritize   Recovery   and Regeneration: Athletic training must include both regeneration and recovery because they help the body adjust to the demands of exercise and gradually enhance performance improvements. Make recovery exercises like foam rolling, stretching, and mobility exercises a priority to release tightness in your muscles, increase your range of motion, and shield yourself from harm. Include dynamic recovery exercises like brisk walking or cycling to increase blood flow, make it easier for nutrients to reach muscles, and improve muscle recovery in between hard training sessions.

Achieving peak performance and optimal fitness on the Carnivore Diet requires a multifaceted approach that integrates exercise, nutrition, and recovery strategies tailored to individual needs and goals. People may achieve optimal fitness on the Carnivore Diet by striking the correct balance between activity and nutrition, improving muscle development and recovery, and putting helpful advice for athletes and active people into practice. These tips and techniques will enable you to succeed and meet your fitness objectives on the Carnivore Diet, regardless of whether you're a competitive athlete, fitness enthusiast, or just trying to become healthier.

Chapter 9

Carnivore Diet for Special Populations

The Carnivore Diet, with its emphasis on animal-based nutrition, has gained popularity as a dietary approach for promoting health and well-being. Applying it to other populations, including women, children, and older adults, calls for careful analysis of each group's specific physiological requirements and developmental milestones. In this chapter, we look at how the Carnivore Diet might affect certain demographics, providing ideas on how to improve health at each age and any stage of life.

Carnivore Diet for Women

Women need specific dietary approaches to promote general health and well-being because of their unique hormonal profiles, reproductive problems, and nutritional demands. For women, the Carnivore Diet offers both possibilities and problems since it requires careful consideration of nutritional intake, hormonal balance, and menstrual health.

Supporting Hormonal Health

Women's health and vitality depend heavily on hormone balance, which affects metabolic processes, mood management, and reproductive function. The Carnivore

Diet's focus on animal fat and protein provides vital nutrients and building blocks for the synthesis and control of hormones. However, since micronutrients like iron, zinc, and B vitamins are so important for hormone production and metabolism, it's essential to make sure you're getting enough of them.

To maximize nutritional intake and promote hormonal health, include nutrient-dense animal foods like red meat, organ meats, and shellfish in the diet. Pay attention to symptoms of hormone imbalance, such as weariness, mood swings, and irregular menstruation cycles, and modify your food plans appropriately. Seeking advice from a medical professional or a qualified dietitian with expertise in women's health might provide tailored direction and assistance.

Addressing Nutrient Needs

Women's nutritional needs are specific, especially throughout important life periods including menopause, breastfeeding, and pregnancy. These particular demands may be met by tailoring the Carnivore Diet to emphasize animal foods high in nutrients and high in vital vitamins, minerals, and amino acids. Include iron-rich foods in your diet, such as red meat and organ meats, to maintain healthy blood and avoid iron deficiency anemia, which is a significant worry for fertile women.

Make sure you consume enough protein throughout pregnancy and breastfeeding to support the growth and development of the fetus, the healing of the mother's tissue, and the production of milk. Omega-3 fatty acids, which are crucial for the development of the embryonic brain, are provided by eating fatty fish like salmon and sardines, which may also lower the risk of postpartum depression. For optimal pregnancy and newborn health outcomes, establish dietary sufficiency by consulting with a healthcare physician or registered dietitian.

Managing Weight and Body Composition

Women often worry about their body composition and weight control, which is impacted by a variety of variables including hormone swings, metabolic rate, and lifestyle choices. A low-carb, high-protein weight-management strategy that encourages satiety, fat reduction, and the maintenance of lean muscle mass is provided by the carnivore diet.

Track your energy intake and output to reach and maintain healthy body composition and weight. To promote metabolic health and reduce cravings, emphasize nutrient-dense, satiating meals like meat, fish, eggs, and dairy products. Combine strength training with aerobic exercise to improve cardiovascular fitness, muscular tone, and general health.

Carnivore Diet for Children and Adolescents

Due to their fast growth and development, children and adolescents need a sufficient diet to maintain their mental, emotional, and physical well-being. For this group, the Carnivore Diet presents special issues that need close attention to growth characteristics, nutritional density, and long-term health consequences.

Ensuring Nutritional Adequacy

For kids and teenagers on the Carnivore Diet, adequate nutrition is crucial since it offers the vital elements needed for healthy growth, development, and general well-being. To satisfy your demands for both macro- and micronutrients, give priority to nutrient-dense animal meals such as meat, fish, poultry, eggs, and dairy products. To guarantee a varied range of nutrients and encourage the best possible health results, include a variety of meals from various animal sources.

Track growth metrics like weight, height, and body mass index (BMI) to determine nutritional health and make sure growth and development are happening in the right places. Address any concerns you may have about development, nutrient intake, or nutritional sufficiency of diet by consulting a doctor or registered dietitian with expertise in pediatric nutrition.

Promoting Healthy Eating Habits

Early adoption of good eating practices establishes the groundwork for long-term health and well-being. Encourage kids and teenagers to try a range of meals derived from animals, play around with tastes and textures, and cultivate a healthy connection with food. Plan, prepare, and cook meals with your kids to help them become more independent, creative, and self-assured eaters.

Stress the value of mindful eating, quantity management, and a balanced diet in promoting general health and preventing disordered eating habits. To help children and adolescents develop good habits and attitudes regarding food, body image, and self-care, provide an example of healthy eating practices and attitudes.

Addressing Growth and Development

Development and growth are dynamic processes that are impacted by dietary, environmental, and genetic variables. The Carnivore Diet offers the vital nutrients required for bone health, muscular growth, immune system function, and cognitive function, all of which contribute to the ideal growth and development of kids and teenagers.

Make sure you are getting enough protein, calcium, vitamin D, and other micronutrients that are important for the development of healthy bones and skeletons. To encourage the development of motor skills, coordination, and social interaction, including physical exercise, outdoor play, and leisure sports. Track developmental milestones and progress to spot any problems early and take appropriate action to promote healthy growth and development.

Carnivore Diet for Older Adults

Due to age, the risk of chronic illness, and changes in metabolism, older persons have particular dietary needs. For this demographic, the Carnivore Diet may be advantageous since it supports metabolic health, preserves muscle mass, and improves cognitive performance. To fulfill the requirements of older persons, it is important to address particular problems and customize nutritional methods.

Encouragement of Metabolic Health

As people age, changes in body composition, hormone control, and metabolism all have an impact on their general health and well-being, making metabolic health more and more crucial. The Carnivore Diet promotes stable blood sugar levels, insulin sensitivity, and fat metabolism by taking a low-carb, high-protein approach to metabolic health.

To evaluate metabolic health and spot any possible problems, monitor blood sugar levels and metabolic indicators including insulin, HbA1c, and fasting glucose. To maximize metabolic function and stop the emergence or progression of metabolic illnesses such as type 2 diabetes, insulin resistance, and metabolic syndrome, dietary patterns should be adjusted as necessary.

Supporting Metabolic Health

An increasing number of older persons are concerned about sarcopenia, or age-related muscle loss, which results in a decline in strength, mobility, and functional independence. The Carnivore Diet provides vital amino acids required for muscle protein synthesis and repair, making it a protein-rich strategy for maintaining muscle mass and strength.

To support muscle maintenance and optimum aging, prioritize your diet of high-quality animal sources of protein, such as meat, fish, poultry, eggs, and dairy products. Use resistance training activities to maintain muscle mass, increase strength, and improve functional ability. Examples of these exercises include bodyweight exercises, resistance bands, and weightlifting.

Supporting Cognitive Function and Brain Health

Memory, cognition, and overall quality of life are all impacted by cognitive function and brain health, which are crucial components of good aging. The Carnivore Diet provides vital nutrients including omega-3 fatty acids, choline, and vitamin B12 that are required for brain construction and function, which may have positive effects on cognitive function and brain health.

Add fatty fish to your diet, such as mackerel, sardines, and salmon, to get the omega-3 fatty acids your brain needs to be healthy and perform cognitively. Incorporate high-nutrient animal foods, such as organ meats, eggs, and dairy products, to meet your needs for choline and vitamin B12, two important nutrients for neurotransmitter production and mental function.

The Carnivore Diet presents unique opportunities and considerations for special populations, including women, children adolescents, and older adults. Through customized nutritional approaches that align with the unique requirements and objectives of distinct populations, people may maximize health results, foster growth and development, and improve general well-being over a range of age groups and life phases. These ideas and insights enable people to fully use the Carnivore Diet's potential for lifetime health and vitality, whether managing hormonal shifts, encouraging children to eat healthily, or supporting optimum aging.

Chapter 10

Supplements and Additional Considerations

While the Carnivore Diet emphasizes the consumption of animal-based foods as the primary source of nutrition, there are instances where supplementation and additional considerations may be necessary to optimize health outcomes. In this thorough chapter, we examine the function of supplements as well as other things people on the Carnivore Diet should think about. This book seeks to give helpful insights and information for sustaining health and well-being on the Carnivore Diet, covering everything from necessary supplements to addressing possible nutritional shortages, tracking health indicators, and speaking with medical specialists.

Essential Supplements for Carnivores

While the Carnivore Diet provides a rich array of nutrients from animal-based foods, there are certain vitamins, minerals, and other supplements that may be beneficial to include in the diet to ensure optimal health and well-being. The vital vitamins for carnivores and their possible contributions to general health support are discussed in this section.

Essential Supplements:

1. Vitamin D: For strong bones, a healthy immune system, and general well-being, vitamin D is necessary. Even though fatty fish and egg yolks are natural sources of vitamin D, some people may need to take supplements, particularly those who live in areas with little sunshine or who don't get enough sun exposure.

2. Omega-3 Fatty Acids: EPA and DHA in particular are essential for brain development, cardiovascular health, and the control of inflammation. Even while fatty fish like salmon and sardines are great providers of omega-3s, those who eat little to no seafood may find that they are getting enough by taking supplements like krill or fish oil.

3. Vitamin B12: Red blood cell development, neurological function, and the synthesis of energy all depend on vitamin B12. Although the main source of vitamin B12 is animal-based foods, people who have restricted diets or those with reduced absorption may need to take supplements.

4. Electrolytes: Important for nerve transmission, muscular contraction, and hydration, electrolytes include sodium, potassium, and magnesium. Even though animal meals include electrolytes, those who are suffering from electrolyte imbalances or who are physically active may benefit from supplements.

5. Creatine: A naturally occurring substance in animal diets, creatine is necessary for the body to produce energy during vigorous activity. Creatine monohydrate supplements may improve muscular strength, power, and performance, especially for those doing resistance training or other high-intensity exercises.

Addressing Potential Nutrient Deficiencies

While the Carnivore Diet provides a nutrient-dense array of animal-based foods, there may be instances where individuals are at risk of nutrient deficiencies due to dietary restrictions, absorption issues, or other factors. The major nutritional shortages in the

Carnivore Diet are discussed in this section along with solutions.

Common Nutrient Deficiencies:

1. Vitamin C: Although meat has trace quantities of this vitamin, a Carnivore Diet may not supply enough to fulfill daily needs. Consider eating organ meats like liver, which are high in vitamin C, to remedy this shortage, or take vitamin C supplements if needed.

2. Fiber: The Carnivore Diet's lack of plant-based meals may lead to a decrease in fiber consumption, which may have an impact on intestinal health and regularity. Even though carnivores usually have fewer digestive problems, constipation may be helped by adding bone broth, collagen powder, or psyllium husk fiber supplements to your diet.

3. Calcium: Dairy products and certain fish with edible bones are good sources of calcium, but those who avoid these meals run the danger of not getting enough of it. To maintain bone health, think about including foods high in calcium, such as canned sardines or fish with bones, or taking supplements of calcium citrate if needed.

4. Iron: Although heme iron, which is highly accessible, is found in red meat, those who consume less meat or have problems with absorption may not get enough iron. To avoid anemia, think about eating foods high in iron, such as chicken, beef liver, or shellfish, or taking iron supplements if needed.

Monitoring Health Markers and Adjusting as Needed

On the Carnivore Diet, maintaining optimum health requires routinely checking important health indicators and making necessary dietary and lifestyle adjustments. This section looks at key health indicators to monitor and methods for maximizing health benefits when following a carnivore diet.

Key Health Markers:

1. Blood Lipids: Tracking lipid profiles, which include lipoprotein particles, triglycerides, and cholesterol levels, may provide information about metabolic and cardiovascular health. Although many people's lipid profiles have been shown to improve with the Carnivore Diet, some people may have temporary increases in cholesterol, especially LDL cholesterol. If necessary, get medical advice from a professional to interpret lipid test findings and choose the best course of action.

2. Blood Sugar Levels: Monitoring HbA1c and fasting blood glucose levels may provide information about metabolic health and glycemic management. Because of its low-carbohydrate content, the Carnivore Diet usually results in stable blood sugar levels and enhanced insulin sensitivity. Nonetheless, those with diabetes or insulin resistance should regularly check their blood sugar levels and, under medical supervision, change their medication dosage as necessary.

3. Micronutrient Status: Frequent evaluation of vitamin and mineral levels, as well as micronutrient status, may help detect any deficiencies and direct the development of supplementing plans. Collaborate with a medical professional or registered dietitian to carry out thorough nutritional testing and create individualized supplement plans depending on food preferences and personal requirements.

4. Inflammatory Markers: Immune function and systemic inflammation may be better understood by keeping an eye on inflammatory markers like interleukin-6 (IL-6) and C-reactive protein (CRP). Individual reactions to dietary changes may differ, even though the Carnivore Diet is naturally low in inflammatory items like processed carbs and vegetable oils. Keep an eye out for signs of inflammation, such as weariness, digestive problems, or joint discomfort, and modify your food and way of life as necessary to reduce inflammation.

Consulting with Healthcare Professionals

To optimize health results and navigate the complexity of the Carnivore Diet, healthcare experts such as doctors, registered dietitians, and other competent practitioners must collaborate. This section discusses the value of getting expert advice and methods for locating medical professionals who support the carnivore diet.

Importance of Professional Guidance:

1. Personalized Nutrition Advice: Based on a patient's dietary choices, medical circumstances, and health objectives, healthcare providers may provide individualized nutrition advice. Whether you're trying to manage chronic conditions, improve sports performance, address vitamin deficiencies, or improve your diet, working with a licensed dietitian or nutritionist may help you create a personalized plan for eating healthy.

2. Monitoring Health Parameters: Medical practitioners can help with routine tracking of vital signs such as blood lipids, blood sugar, and vitamin status. Practitioners may evaluate the success of dietary treatments, spot possible health hazards, and provide well-informed recommendations to maximize health outcomes by monitoring these indicators over time.

3. Addressing Potential Risks: Although the Carnivore Diet may be beneficial for a large number of people, it may not be appropriate for everyone, particularly for those who have particular dietary needs or underlying medical concerns. When it comes to the Carnivore Diet, medical specialists may assist in identifying possible hazards and contraindications as well as provide advice on other dietary methods and supplementation procedures.

4. Long-Term Health Planning: Taking into account nutritional, lifestyle, and medical issues necessitates a comprehensive approach to long-term health and well-being planning. To support the best possible health results on the Carnivore Diet, healthcare experts may assist in the development of sustainable dietary regimens, treat any nutritional shortages, and provide continuous support and advice.

Supplementation and additional considerations play a crucial role in optimizing health outcomes for individuals following the Carnivore Diet. These measures allow people to maintain health and well-being on the Carnivore Diet by addressing any nutritional shortages, monitoring health indicators, and consulting with healthcare specialists, in addition to providing vital supplements. People may confidently negotiate the complexity of the Carnivore Diet and achieve excellent long-term health results by working with skilled practitioners, monitoring important health metrics, and giving tailored nutrition recommendations priority.

Chapter 11

Troubleshooting and FAQs

Embarking on the Carnivore Diet journey can bring transformative health benefits, but it's not without its challenges and questions. We cover frequent roadblocks, moral dilemmas, and pressing inquiries that people may have while implementing the Carnivore Diet in this extensive manual. With a focus on sustainability, ethics, and frequently asked questions, this book attempts to provide readers with the information and tools necessary to successfully and confidently traverse their carnivore journey.

Common Challenges and Solutions

There may be some difficulties while switching to a carnivore diet since the body will need time to adjust to the new eating pattern. This section examines typical problems that carnivores face and provides workable answers.

Common Challenges:

1. Transition Period: As the body gets used to consuming less carbohydrates, some people may feel discomfort during the early phase of the Carnivore Diet. This discomfort may include headaches, lethargy, and digestive problems. Known as the "keto flu," this transitional phase usually ends in a few days to weeks as the body adjusts to becoming fat-adapted.

2. Digestive Issues: Although many people handle the carnivore diet well, some people may have digestive problems such as bloating, diarrhea, or constipation. Changes in the amount of fiber consumed, the makeup of the gut bacteria, or dehydration may all contribute to these problems. Digestion pain may be reduced by drinking more water, adding collagen powder or bone broth, and experimenting with various meat cuts and cooking techniques.

3. Social Challenges: Eating a carnivore diet may be socially challenging, especially when eating out with loved ones or in public. To overcome these obstacles and adhere to dietary preferences and health objectives, it might be helpful to address worries about social acceptability, cultural standards, and dietary limitations. Openly discuss your dietary preferences with close ones, volunteer to bring carnivore-friendly meals to get-togethers, and put more emphasis on the people than the food.

4. Cravings and Food Temptations: During the early phases of a diet or in reaction to emotional stimuli, cravings for non-carnivore foods may surface. To control cravings and stick to dietary plans, try mindful eating, identifying your hunger triggers, and finding enjoyable carnivore-friendly substitutes. Try varying meat cuts, cooking methods, and spices to add variety and satisfaction to your meals.

Addressing Concerns About Sustainability and Ethics

Because the carnivore diet places a strong focus on items derived from animals, concerns over its sustainability and ethics are widespread. This section addresses these issues and offers suggestions on how people might adopt a sustainable and morally sound approach to the carnivore diet.

Sustainability Considerations:

1. Regenerative Agriculture: Adopting regenerative agricultural techniques may improve soil health, biodiversity, and carbon sequestration while reducing negative environmental effects. Seek animal products from ranches and farms that value regenerative methods like pasture-raised crops, rotational grazing, and comprehensive land management.

2. Nose-to-Tail Eating: By using whole animals and reducing waste, adopting this eating style supports sustainability. To optimize nutritional variety and reduce environmental impact, include cuts high in collagen, organ meats, and bones in your diet. Try different recipes and cooking methods to include less often eaten animal parts.

3. Local and Sustainable Sourcing: Reducing the carbon footprint related to food production and transportation may be achieved by promoting local farmers and sustainable food systems. To reduce your influence on the environment and help small-scale farmers, look for locally produced animal products at farmers' markets, via community-supported agriculture (CSA) programs, or through farm-to-table efforts.

Ethical Considerations:

1. Animal Welfare: At the core of ethical carnivory is the prioritization of animal welfare, which guarantees that animals get humane treatment and are grown in conditions that support their natural behaviors and general well-being. Select animal products from ranches and farms that uphold strict guidelines for animal welfare, such as those who rear their animals on pastures, feed them grass, and don't use hormones.

2. Respectful Consumption: This approach recognizes the sacrifice made by the animals that provide us with our food and shelter. Thank the farmers who grow the animals and the animals themselves, and try to reduce waste by using all of the animal's components and devouring it in moderation.

3. Ethical Hunting and Fishing: Sustainable harvests and respect for wildlife populations are ensured by ethical hunting and fishing methods for individuals who choose to include wild game or fish in their diet. Respect local laws and ordinances, hunt and fish ethically, and give conservation efforts priority to protect ecosystems and natural habitats.

FAQs: Answering Your Burning Questions

Addressing common questions and concerns can provide clarity and guidance for individuals navigating the Carnivore Diet journey. To assist people in making educated dietary decisions, this section answers often-asked questions and offers evidence-based responses.

FAQs:

1. Is the Carnivore Diet safe for long-term health?

When the individual's health demands, nutritional diversity, and enough intake of nutrients are taken into consideration, the Carnivore Diet may be safe and sustainable for long-term health. To make sure your diet is enough, speak with a doctor or certified nutritionist. You should also routinely check your health indicators.

2. Will I miss out on essential nutrients by eliminating plant foods?

Foods derived from animals include vital minerals, such as protein, iron, zinc, vitamin B12, and omega-3 fatty acids, in highly accessible forms. People may achieve their nutritional demands on the Carnivore Diet by emphasizing nutrient-dense animal products and including a range of cuts and sources.

3. Can I still achieve fitness and athletic goals on the Carnivore Diet?

By providing the high-quality protein, vital amino acids, and healthy fats required for muscle repair, recovery, and energy generation, the carnivore diet may enhance physical fitness and performance. To maximize athletic objectives, try out various training methods, track performance indicators, and make necessary nutritional adjustments.

4. What about cholesterol and heart health?

Research indicates that the Carnivore Diet may enhance lipid profiles overall by boosting HDL cholesterol and lowering triglycerides and LDL particle size, even if it may cause temporary rises in cholesterol for certain people. To maximize heart health, speak with a healthcare professional about monitoring cholesterol levels and making any dietary adjustments.

Navigating challenges and answering questions on the Carnivore Diet journey requires a combination of practical solutions, ethical considerations, evidence-based information, and community support. This guide aims to empower people to thrive on their carnivore journey with confidence, clarity, and success by addressing common challenges, answering commonly asked questions, addressing sustainability and ethical concerns, and providing resources for more information and support.